Coconut Oil Beauty Secrets

You Wish You Knew

Disclaimer

"Coconut Oil Beauty Secrets" – At a Glance

We are constantly looking for the next best and greatest one stop beauty solution. Products that will make us look younger and healthier. We throw loads of money in salons in spas trying to get the best possible look because seriously, who doesn't want to look good? But what if I told you that you can save all that precious hard earned money because there is something in your kitchen right now that can help you achieve all that? Unbelievable? Not anymore!

Coconut oil is the one stop solution that I am talking about. In this book you will find how coconut oil can enhance your hair growth and help you manage frizzy hair. I will also tell you how coconut oil can become the cure of most of your skin problems ranging from acne to wrinkles. And last but not the least I will share with you how coconut oil is not only good for your outward image but is also great for your heart and health.

This is just the tip of the iceberg. Read along and get mesmerized at how coconut oil can help you achieve great health and improved looks in no time.

Contents

Introduction

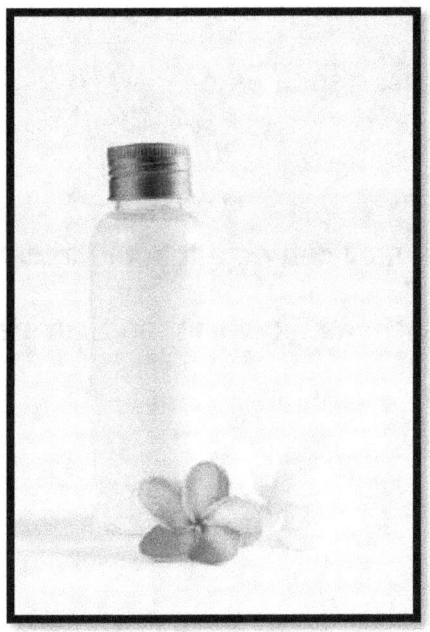

Coconut oil is extracted from the meat or kernel of mature coconuts and is edible. It can be used for a variety of purposes such as in cooking, application on hair and skin, and in medicines.

It is used extensively in tropical countries like the Philippines, Thailand, Sri Lanka, India, etc. Health benefits that you can achieve by using coconut oil include regulated metabolism, improvement in digestion, enhanced immunity, weight loss, maintenance of cholesterol, stress relief, skin care, and hair care.

If these benefits were not enough to get you hooked on coconut oil then let me tell you that coconut oil also plays a vital role in improving your bone strength, and dental quality. It also helps with various diseases such as cancer, HIV, diabetes, high blood pressure, heart diseases and kidney problems.

All of these qualities for coconut oil can be attributed to caprylic acid, capric acid, lauric acid and their properties; such as soothing and antibacterial qualities, anti-fungal properties, antioxidant, and antimicrobial properties.

Coconut Oil – Composition

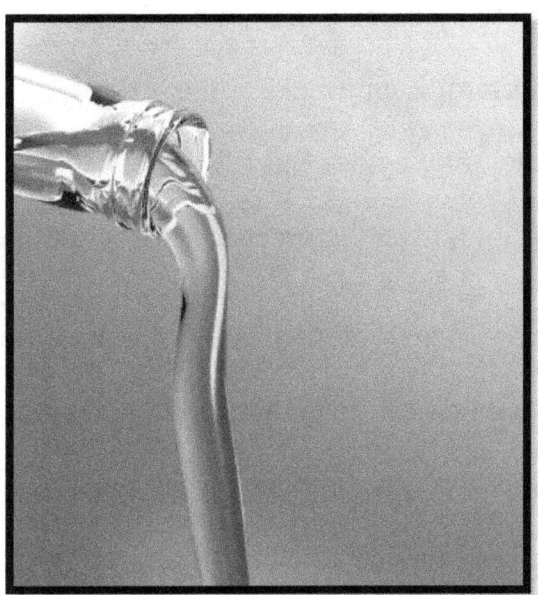

Coconut oil contains many nutrients and minerals. A more detailed analysis of nutrients present in coconut oil will come in a later part of the book but following are the main components of coconut oil:

Poly-Phenols

Coconuts have Gallic acid, also called Phenolic acid. This acid is responsible for the fragrance and taste of virgin coconut oil and coconut oil.

Monounsaturated Fatty Acids

Coconut oil contains Oleic acid.

Polyunsaturated Fatty Acids

Coconut oil also contains Linoleic acid.

Saturated Fatty Acids

The majority of the saturated acids in coconut oil are triglycerides that are easily assimilated in the blood stream. Lauric acid is the main component and makes up for about 40 percent of the total fatty acids. Palmitic acid, Myristic acid, Caprylic acid, and Capric acid are also important fatty acids present in coconut oil.

Coconut oil also contains some derivatives of fatty acids like polyol esters, monoglyscerides, fatty polysorbates, fatty ethoxylates, ethanolamide, and betaines. It also contains some derivates of fatty alcohols like fatty alcohol ether sulphate, fatty alcohol sulphate, and fatty chlorides. Vitamin K, Vitamin E and minerals such as Iron are also present in coconut oil.

Types of Coconut Oil

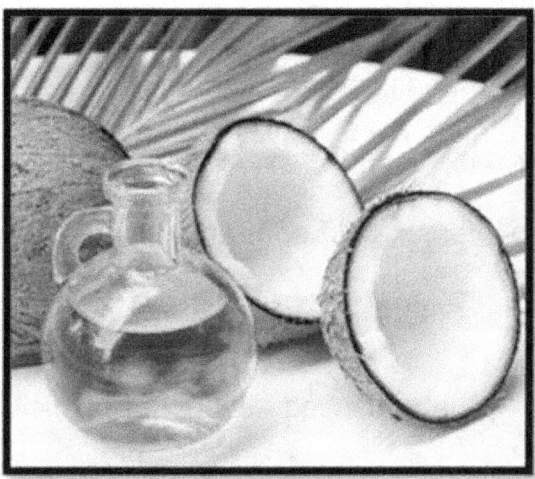

Coconut oil is available in two varieties; refined and unrefined. Both of these types have their own advantages.

Refined

Refined coconut oil has been deodorized and bleached. It is derived from the meal of the coconut, also called copra. The oil obtained from copra needs to be purified through bleaching clays because copra might get contaminated during the drying process. To remove the distinct flavor and odor of coconut oil it is deodorized on high heat.

After refining, coconut oil become fairly tasteless and odorless. Since it is deodorized on high heat it can withstand cooking at high temperatures which makes it an ideal oil for deep frying without adding any coconut flavor to the food item that you are frying in it.

Unrefined

Unrefined coconut oil is usually labeled as extra-virgin or virgin. It is extracted from the fresh, raw coconut without the addition of any chemicals. Depending on the method that has been used to extract the oil, the odor and flavor of unrefined coconut oil remains intact and can range from mild to intense. Mild odor and flavor in coconut oil is a proof of high quality virgin coconut oil.

Since unrefined coconut oil is unprocessed it is more beneficial for your health. You can use it for cooking or apply it on your skin and hair. It can also be used as an ingredient in soap and lotion, massage oil, dietary supplements, syrups, and smoothies.

Now that we have a basic knowledge about coconut oil let us look into its nutritional value.

Coconut Oil – Nutritional Information

The main constituent of coconut oil is Lauric acid which is made up of medium-chain fatty acids. There are numerous health advantages of fatty acids such as:

1. It boosts the immune system

2. It has anticancer qualities

3. It is antibacterial

4. It is antiviral

Whether the coconut oil is unrefined or refined, both are rich in this type of acid. However, unrefined coconut oil is richer in phytonutrients than oil that has been refined. Due to the fact that when coconut oil is bleached and deodorized at high heat, polyphenols which are antioxidants get damaged in the refining process. Therefore unrefined coconut oil is a source of more nutritional elements and from a health standpoint more beneficial than refined.

Part 1 – Coconut Oil for Hair

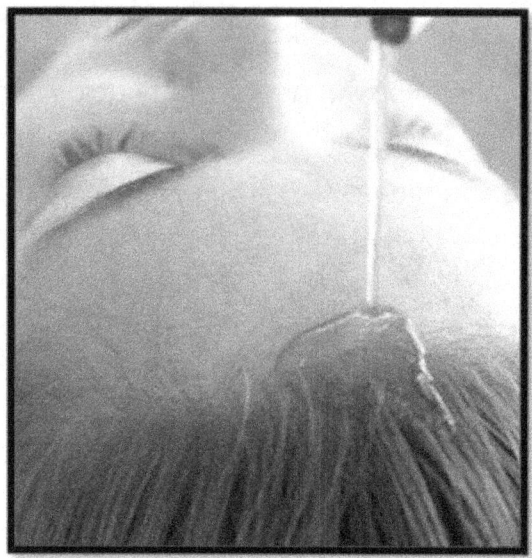

A scalp full of lustrous, shiny and thick hair is a dream for all women, and they can go to great lengths to achieve just that. You can buy the best and most expensive products and spend hundreds of dollars in salon treatments and still might not get the results that you are looking for. But what if I told you that getting healthy, shiny and beautiful hair is not as hard as it looks and you can achieve beautiful hair just by using coconut oil? Shocking isn't it? But totally possible!

For thousands of years coconut oil has been one of the most famous and popular hair conditioners used by tropical countries. Not only does it improve the health of your scalp and enhance your hair cuticles; but it can also repair the damage that you do to your hair every day. It has antifungal properties that cure dandruff and eliminate the need for throwing money away on expensive dandruff shampoos.

In this section I will discuss how coconut oil can help you with hair growth, what the best way of applying coconut oil to your hair is and the added benefits that you can attain by switching to coconut oil.

Hair Growth

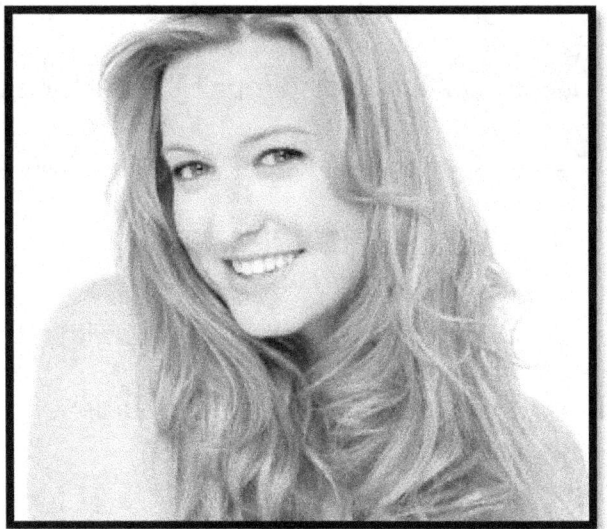

The growth of your hair is influenced by a lot of factors. It is not only about what you apply on your hair but it is also about what you eat and the kind of surroundings that your hair is exposed to. A vast majority of women think that using expensive products is going to do it all, but this is not the case. You need to tend to your hair and take care of it not just drown it in heavily processed products that are loaded with chemicals that might be doing your hair more harm than good.

I understand that you have a very busy schedule and that taking out time for yourself is usually not possible. In order to achieve beautiful, long and healthy hair you need to institute and follow a good hair care regimen that includes an application of oil in your hair. Below are some examples of the ways in which coconut oil promotes hair growth.

Locks Hair Protein

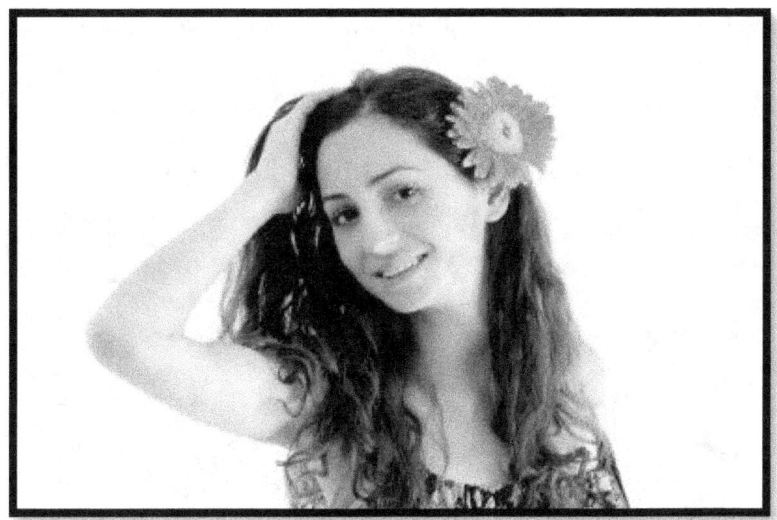

Fatty acids present in coconut oil bind to the protein present in our hair. It protects the overall health of your hair from root to tip. Coconut oil contains Lauric acid which gives better results than any other oils available (such as sunflower oil) to promote healthy hair.

Preserves Moisture

Oiling your hair on a regular basis is a perfect way for retaining the moisture of your hair. Coconut oil penetrates the hair shaft and protects the roots against impurities and excess heat.

Enhances Circulation of Blood

Massaging coconut oil into your hair will enhance the circulation of blood to the scalp area and boost delivery of oxygen and nutrients to your hair.

A Perfect Source of Nutrition

Coconut oil contains nutrients and antioxidants which provide resources that are essential to enhance the luster and shine of your hair. It is also rich in Iron, Vitamin E, and Vitamin K that helps in getting rid of dandruff and boost hair growth at the same time.

Possess Antifungal and Antibacterial Properties

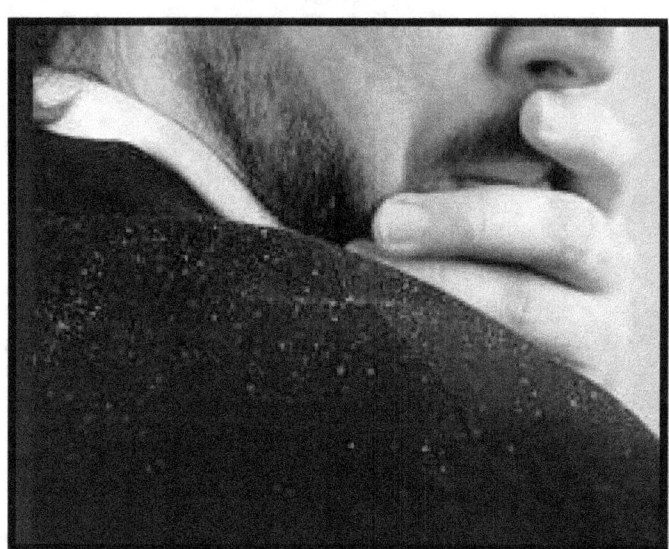

The hair and scalp usually contain elevated levels of bacterial content due to exposure to hazardous environmental factors. Coconut oil is one of the best remedies available to treat and eliminate this issue. Coconut oil provides both antibacterial and antifungal properties that when applied, will protect your hair and scalp against possible outbreaks of lice and dandruff.

Benefits of Coconut Oil

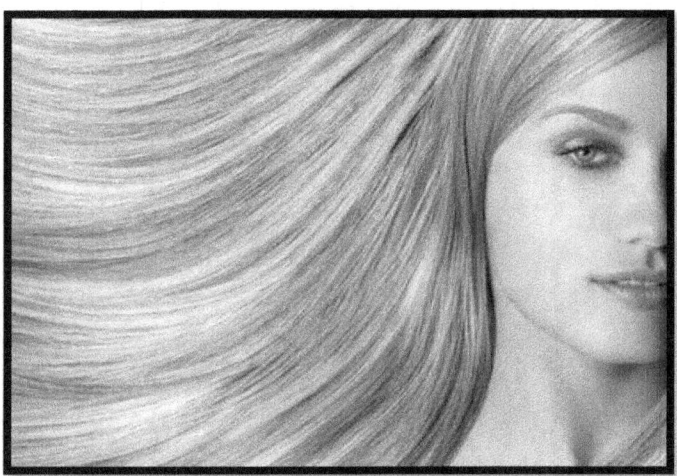

Some of the most important benefits from applying coconut oil in your hair:

1. Coconut oil is a perfect remedy for common scalp complaints and dandruff.

2. It has a prolonged shelf life which means that you can use it over an extended period of time unlike normal hair care products.

3. It is also perfect for conditioning hair.

4. Regular application of coconut oil keeps hair healthy, strong and shiny.

5. It contains Vitamin E which rebuilds and retains hair protein that is lost due to hair styling such as curling or straightening.

6. It has a very nice tropical and lush fragrance which will help your hair smell good too.

How to Apply Coconut Oil on Hair

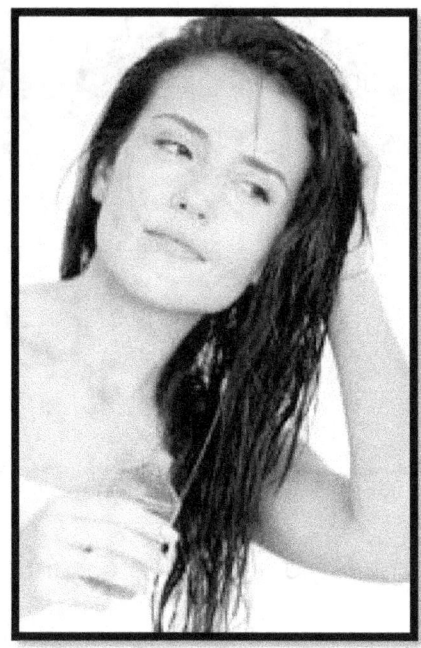

The most important consideration when applying oil to hair is that no impurities or other additives should be added to it. You will obtain the best results by using only coconut oil. These are the steps for applying coconut oil in your hair:

1. Warm Oil

Place the jar of coconut oil in warm water and allow it to heat for a while. Coconut oil usually appears as a white solid at room temperature but melts when you place it in warm water. Make sure that you don't place it in the microwave as that might alter the chemical properties of the oil.

2. Dampen Hair with Warm Water

Thoroughly dampen your hair with slightly warm water before applying coconut oil.

3. Spoon Oil

Take one tablespoon of coconut oil and pour it into the palm of your hand. Begin to apply it directly to the roots of your hair. The ideal amount of oil to apply in your hair is about 2 tablespoons if you have hair that reaches your shoulder and 4 tablespoon if you have longer hair. Use your fingertips to apply coconut oil directly to the scalp and roots of your hair.

4. Massage Gently

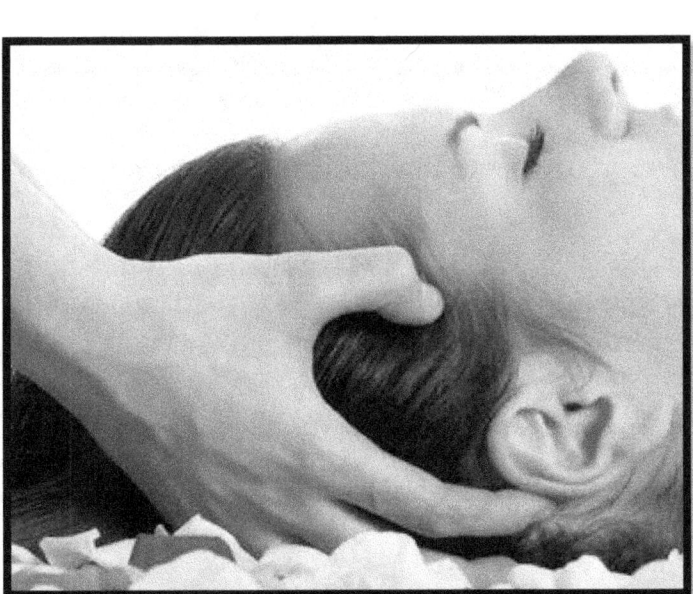

Gently massage your roots for at least 3 minutes to get the best possible results while enhancing the circulation of blood to your scalp. Don't fret if a few strands of hair fall out because that is normal while you are massaging your scalp.

5. Use a Shower Cap

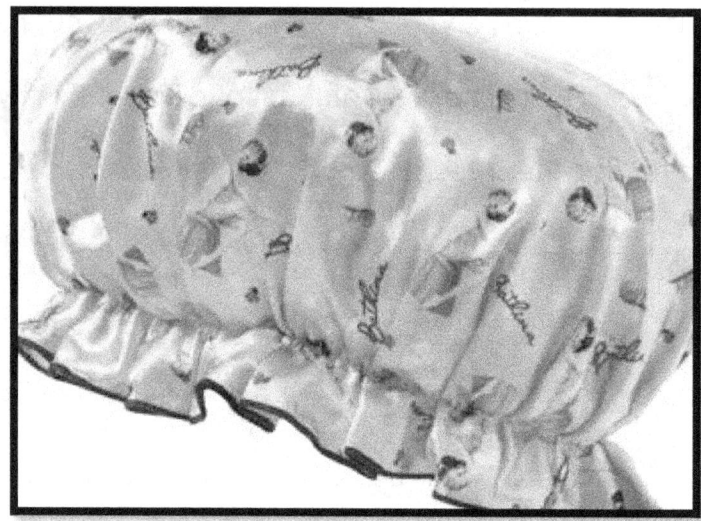

Place a shower cap over your hair so that the coconut oil can get to your roots and work its magic.

6. Wait

Wait for at least 20 to 30 minutes after applying oil. If you have more time that you can leave it in for an hour or two, that would allow for the coconut oil to get thoroughly absorbed in your scalp.

7. Wash It Off

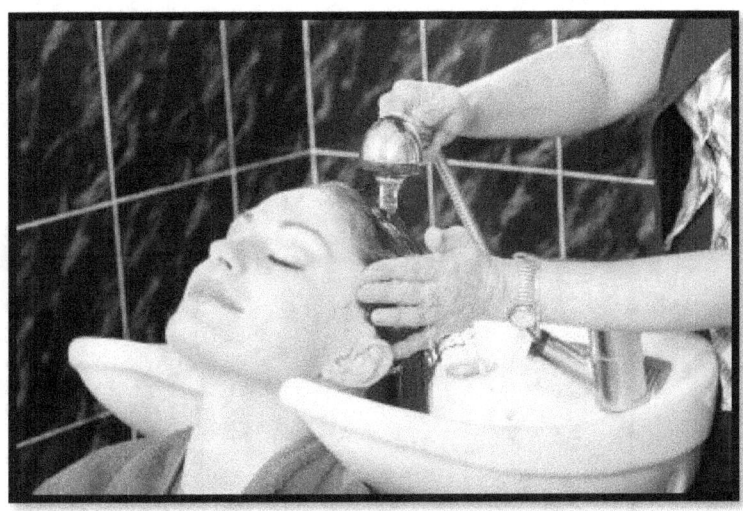

Gently rinse your hair with your shampoo, preferably one that is sulfate free. After applying coconut oil the need to apply conditioner will be nonexistent as it will leave your hair silky, shiny and soft.

Part 2 – Coconut Oil for Skin

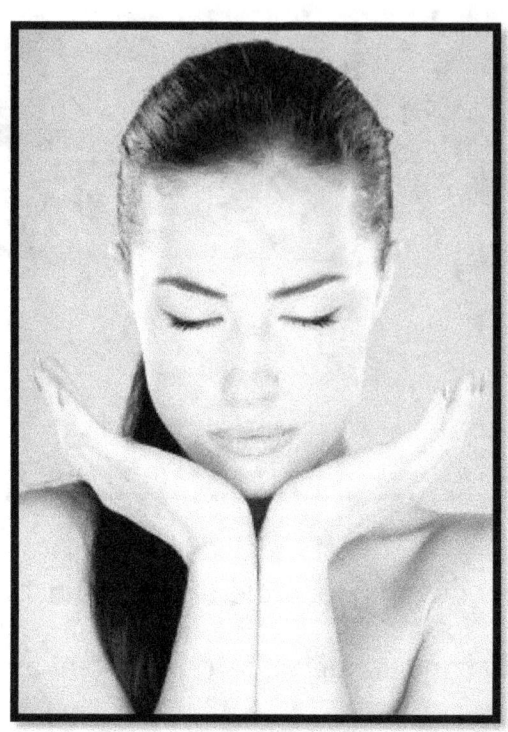

Don't you just love buying products that can provide you with healthy and radiant skin? What you didn't know is that there is an amazing beauty product in one of your kitchen cupboards! That miraculous product is coconut oil.

Coconut oil is extremely good for skin. It contains saturated fats, most of which are in the form of medium chains of triglycerides which are short sections of healthy fat that does not get stored and can be quickly used by the body for energy.

In this section I will discuss how coconut oil can be an answer to solving your various skin problems. As well as how it can benefit you and what are the ways in which you can apply coconut oil on your skin.

One Stop Beauty Treatment

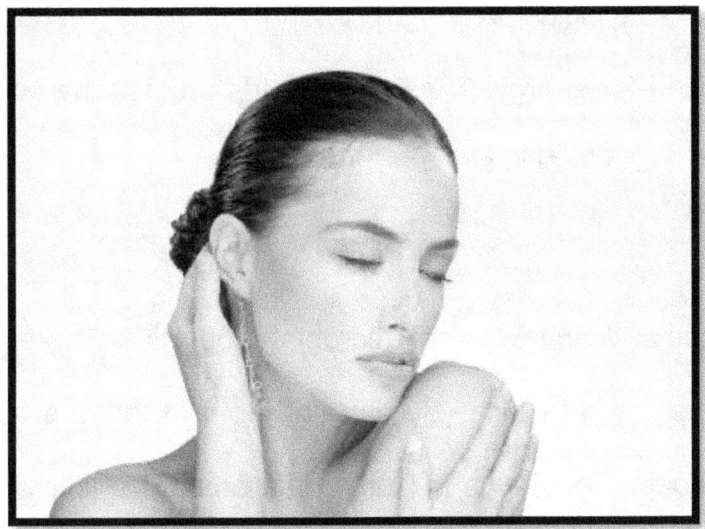

Following are some of the most important ways in which coconut oil can be used to enhance the health of your skin.

Moisturizer

Coconut oil has a high capacity for retaining moisture; so when it is applied to the skin it locks the moisture in your skin and makes it soft and supple.

Emollient

Fatty acids present in coconut oil act as an emollient giving your skin a soothing and softening effect. Small wounds caused by pimples and acne are healed more rapidly than with no treatment. It also helps alleviate dry skin and itchiness and is very effective for people who suffer from psoriasis, eczema, and dermatitis.

It Nourishes the Skin

The medium chains of fatty acids present in coconut oil are absorbed in skin easily where they are directly utilized for energy. These fatty acids provide the energy that is needed by the skin to maintain and heal itself.

Antimicrobial and Antiseptic

Coconut oil possesses antiseptic and antimicrobial properties. There are hardly any FDA approved drugs in the market which you can find both of these properties at the same time in the same product. This helps in limiting the amount of microbes that are able to grow on your skin. In addition this helps to cleanse your skin from various conditions like eczema, dermatitis, and psoriasis and various other skin infections that can cause your skin to look dull, blemished, or aged.

Acne Treatment

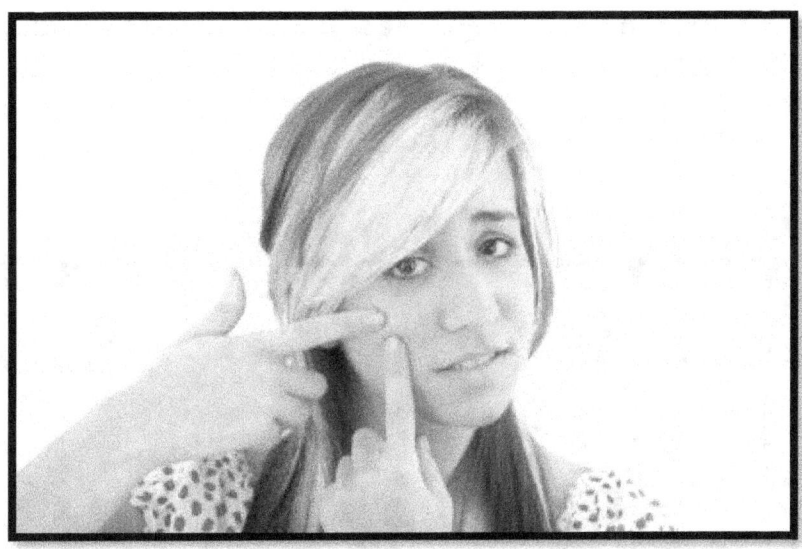

Acne is caused by bacteria called acne vulgaris and coconut oil has the ability to kill this bacteria. Steam your face and then apply a very thin layer of coconut oil on your skin for about 2 minutes and carefully wipe it off. Make sure that you don't leave it on your skin for too long as it might clog your pores and increase the problem.

Antioxidant

Our skin needs antioxidants to fight the free radicals present on its surface. P-coumaric acid and ferulic acid are two main antioxidants present in coconut oil that can help to reduce the free radicals in your skin and leave your skin looking fresher, younger and wrinkle free.

Massage oil

Coconut oil gets absorbed in the skin very easily and therefore makes a perfect oil for body massage.

Natural Deodorant

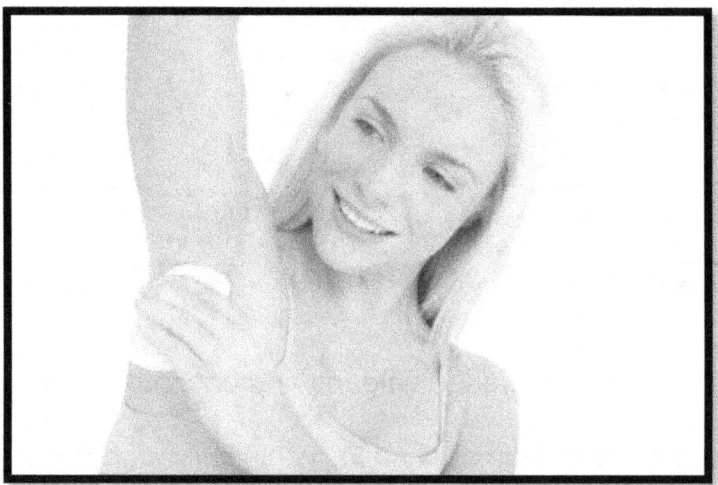

Coconut oil contains properties that can kill microbes and is therefore a perfect remedy of bad body odor because it is caused by bacterial growth. Applying coconut oil under your arms can make a huge difference.

Uses of Coconut Oil

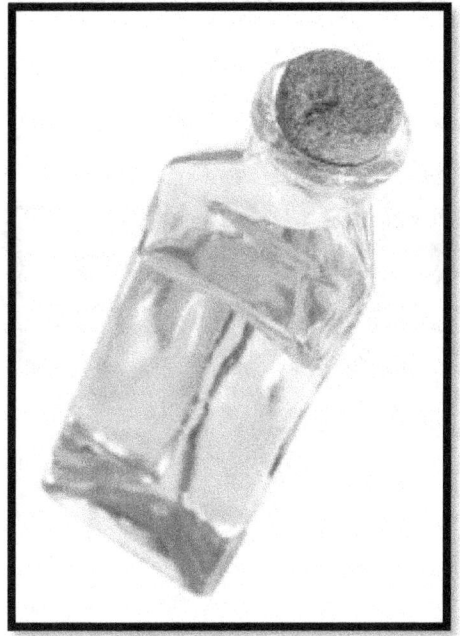

Following are some of the ways in which you can add coconut oil to your skin care regimen to enhance your skin and save some hard earned bucks on expensive beauty products.

Makeup Remover

Place some coconut oil on a cotton pad and rub it gently on your face in circles. It will cleanse your skin gently and smoothly without exposing it to harmful and abrasive chemicals present in normal makeup removers. Make sure that you wash your face after removing your makeup with coconut oil so it does not clog pores.

Shaving Cream

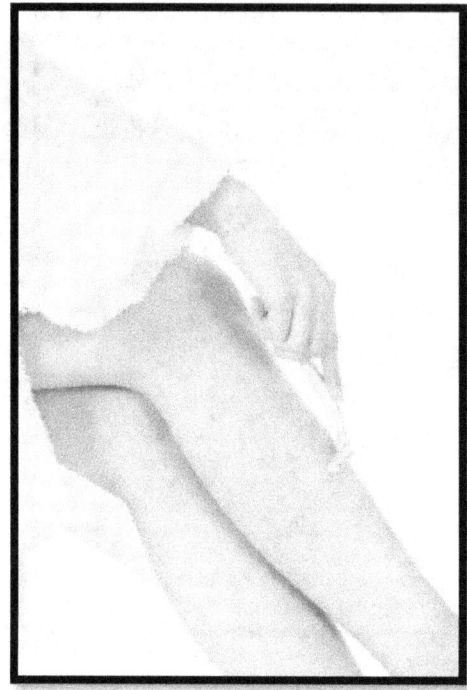

Substitute your shaving cream with coconut oil and see the difference in your skin. This is a great alternative of shaving creams for people who are sensitive to the chemicals that are usually found in shaving creams.

Moisturizer

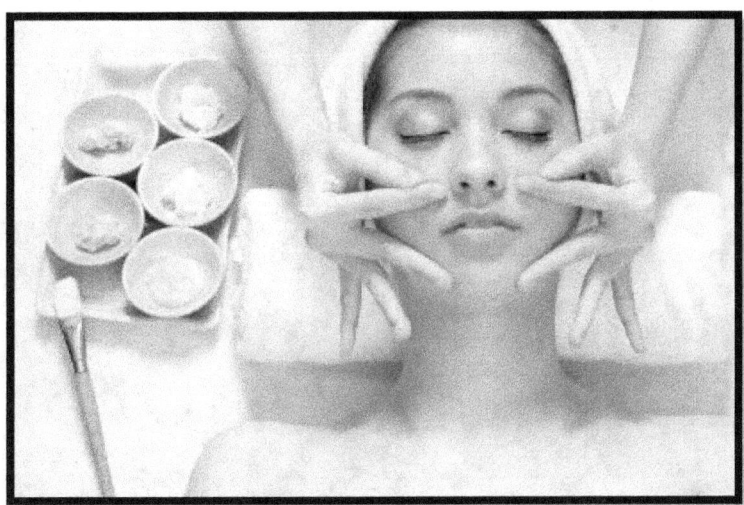

Fatty acids present in coconut oil helps in locking the moisture in your skin. You can apply coconut oil to rough elbows and other dry or rough spots to heal and soften the skin.

Body Scrub

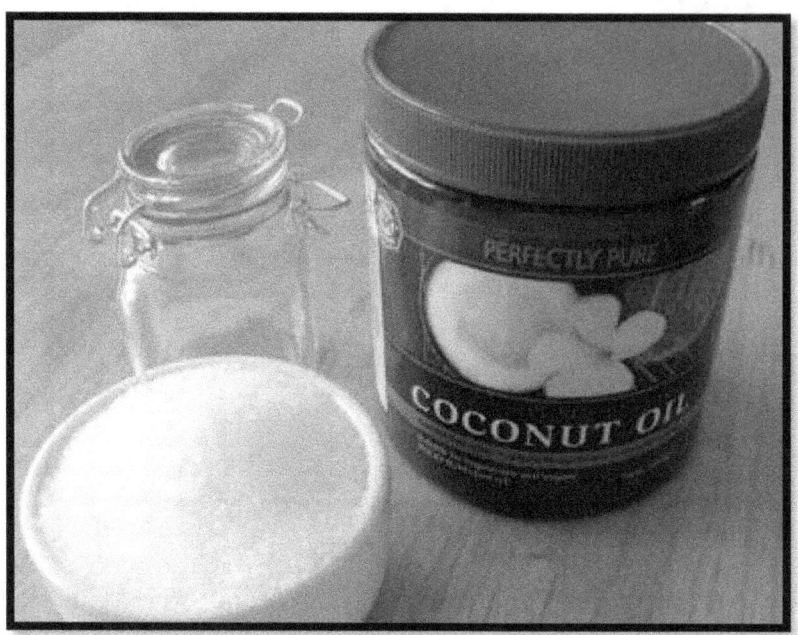

Combine sugar and coconut oil to make your very own body scrub without any added chemicals. Its antifungal properties make it ideal as a foot scrub also.

Face Scrub

To make a face exfoliator, mix a little baking soda in coconut oil and apply it on your face as a scrub.

Face Wash

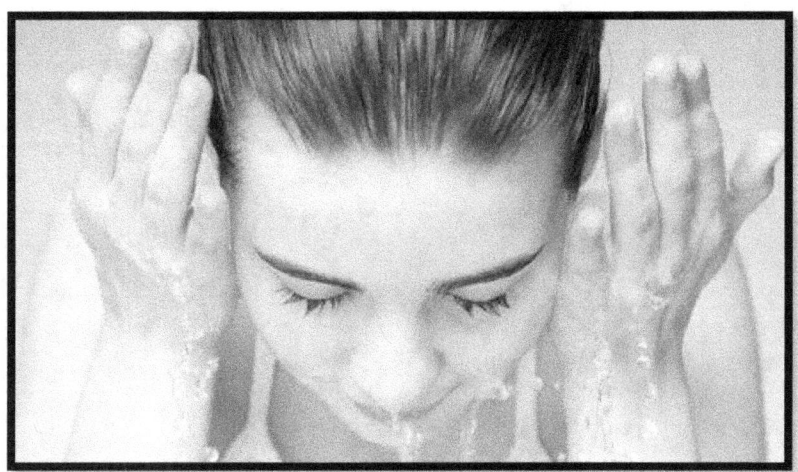

Replace your normal face wash with coconut oil and experience a clearer, smoother and healthier skin.

Eye Cream

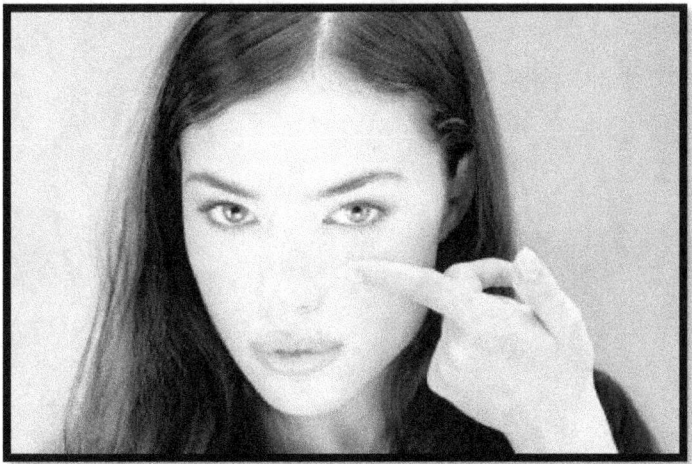

The area around your eyes is most prone to getting wrinkled. Apply coconut oil around your eyes to get a wrinkle free and baby soft skin.

How to Apply Coconut Oil on Skin

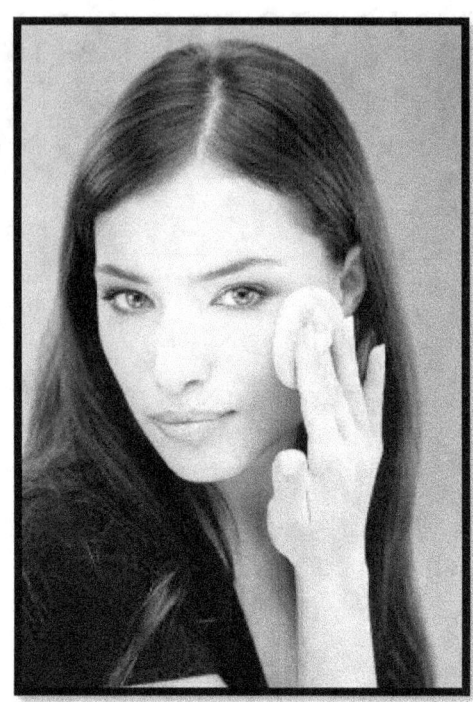

Applying coconut oil on your skin is very easy. Following are some of the ways in which you can apply coconut oil on your face and body.

Face

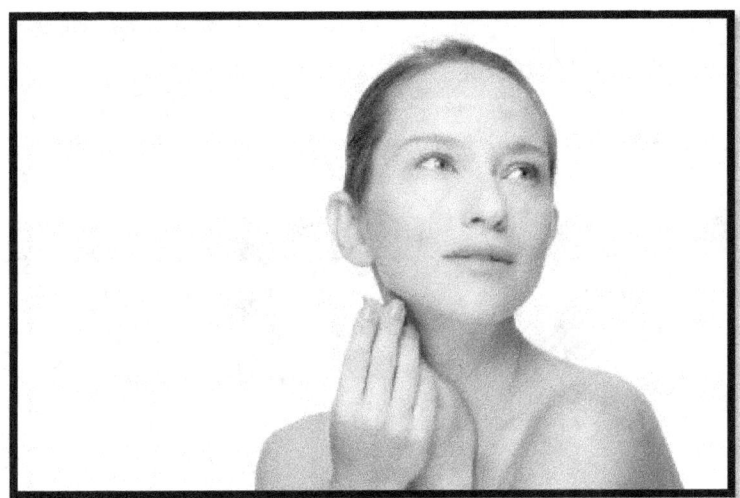

Start with normally washing your face with a face wash or just a splash of water. Use a towel to pat dry your face gently. Once your face is dry, take a little coconut oil and apply it around your eyes. Using a pea size amount of coconut oil for each eye is more than enough and make sure that it does not get in your eyes. If you have other dry areas on your face such as between your eyebrows or other parts of your face then apply a little coconut oil in those areas too. Rub coconut oil gently on the dry patch in a circular motion.

If you have chapped or dry lips, then unrefined coconut oil is the best remedy for moisturizing. Since coconut oil is completely edible, you don't have to worry about ingesting it.

Body

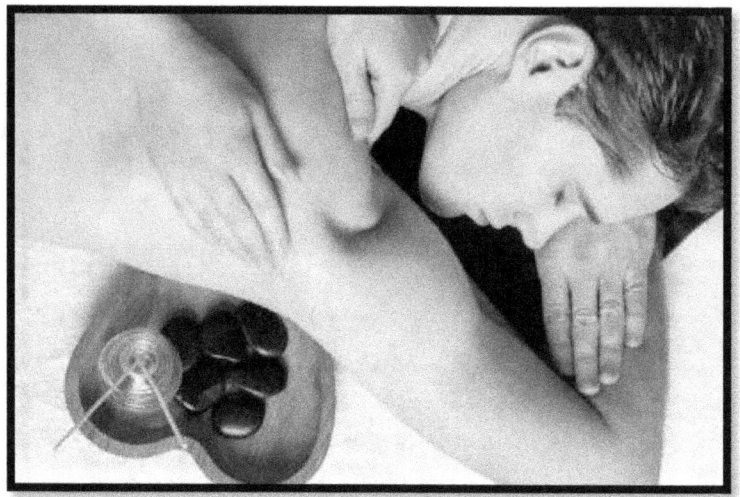

To moisturize your body with coconut oil, apply it on your skin after a shower. Since your skin will be suppler after a shower, the oil will get more readily absorbed and will be more effective.

To moisturize the dry skin areas of your arms, use about a tablespoon of coconut oil and rub it on your arms until it melts from the warmth of your skin. Keep rubbing it on your arms until it is all absorbed in your skin and then repeat the process with the other arm. You can also apply coconut oil on your feet, lower legs, knee areas and thighs in the same way. Moisturize your torso region, by applying coconut oil to your stomach, buttocks, back and breasts. In short you can apply coconut oil on your entire body just like any other skin cream minus the harmful chemicals and additives that are usually found in commercial skin care products.

Part 3 – Coconut Oil for Health

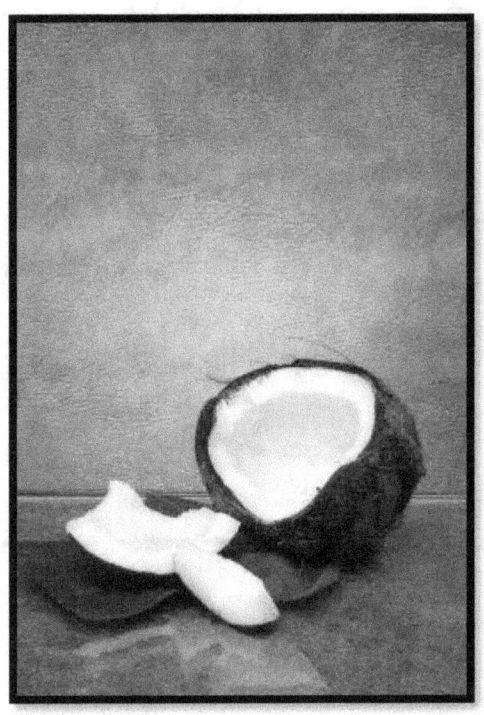

There are only a few food items that can be termed as super foods and coconut oil is one of them. It contains a distinct combination of fatty acids which will help you in achieving a healthier lifestyle.

The health benefits of coconut oil include enhanced brain function and fat loss and a variety of other health benefits that I will be discussing in this section of the book.

Top 10 Health Benefits Of Coconut Oil

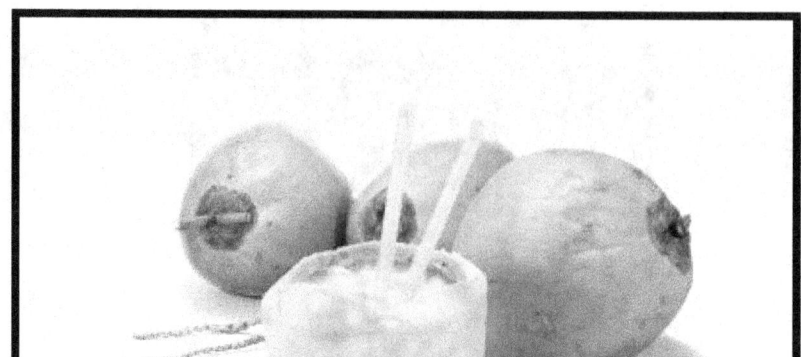

Following are the 10 health benefits that you can obtain by adding coconut oil in to your daily routine.

It Contain Fatty Acids with Effective Medicinal Properties

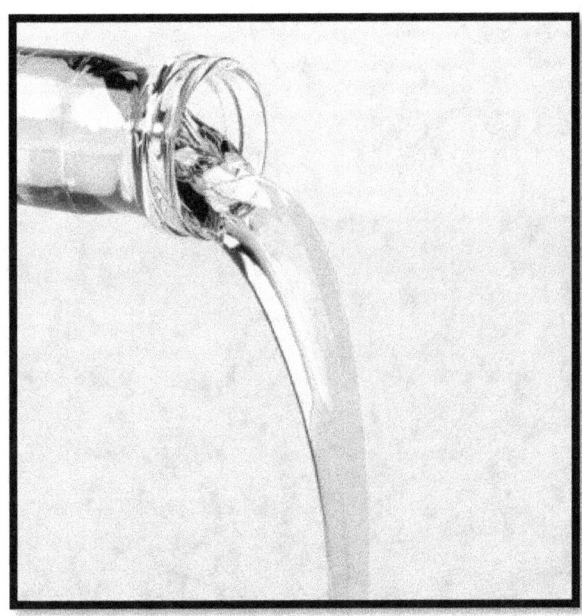

Coconut oil is 90% fatty acids however, these fatty acids are not the harmful kind of saturated fats. Rather they are medium chain triglycerides (MCTs) that are medium length fatty acids. These fatty acids go directly to the digestive tract where they are used instantly to get energy for various body functions. They then turn into ketone bodies that can help with brain disorders like Alzheimer's and epilepsy.

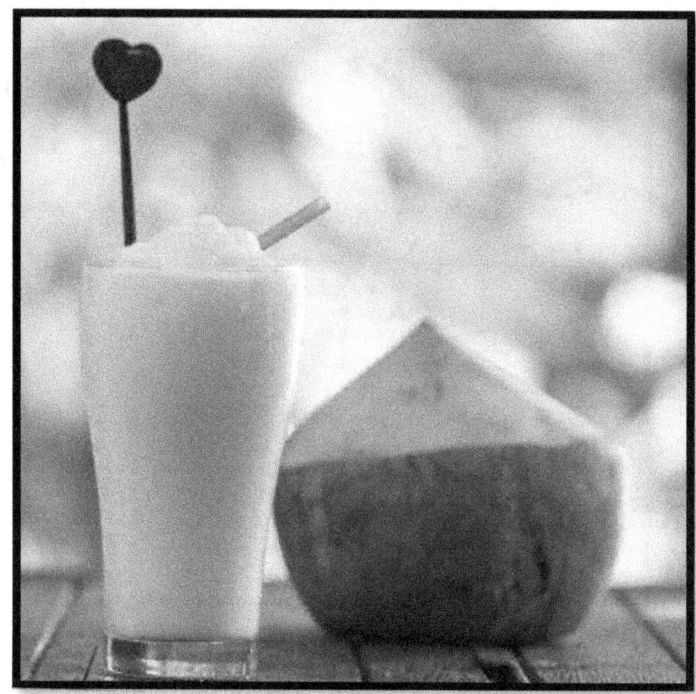

There are many parts of the world where coconut is heavily consumed and is a dietary staple. People have been thriving on it for generations. For example, the population of Tokelauans get 60% of their calories from coconut. The majority of these people have no evidence of heart diseases and are in excellent shape.

It Helps You Burn More Fat

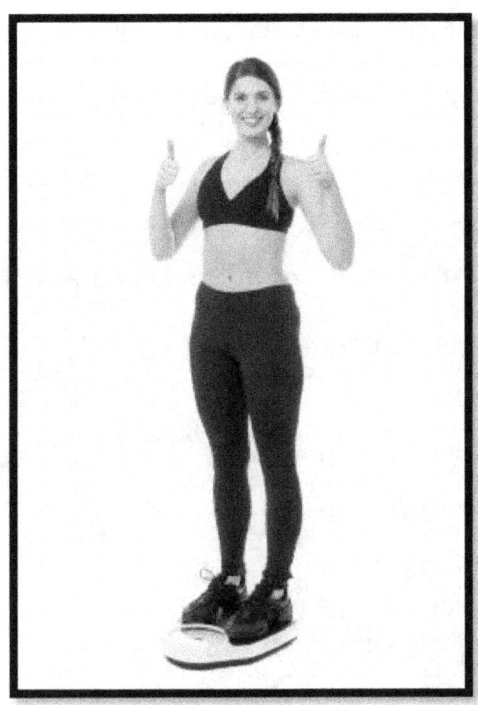

The fatty acids in coconut oil increase the expenditure of energy by 5% which burns fats and helps in weight loss with regular use.

Coconut Oil Kills Bacteria and Saves Us from Fungi and Viruses

Fifty percent of the fatty acids present in coconut oil are Lauric acid. A monoglyceride called monolaurin is formed when coconut oil is digested enzymatically. Both monolaurin and Lauric acid kill dangerous pathogens like fungi, viruses, and bacteria.

Coconut Is the Best Way of Killing Untimely Hunger

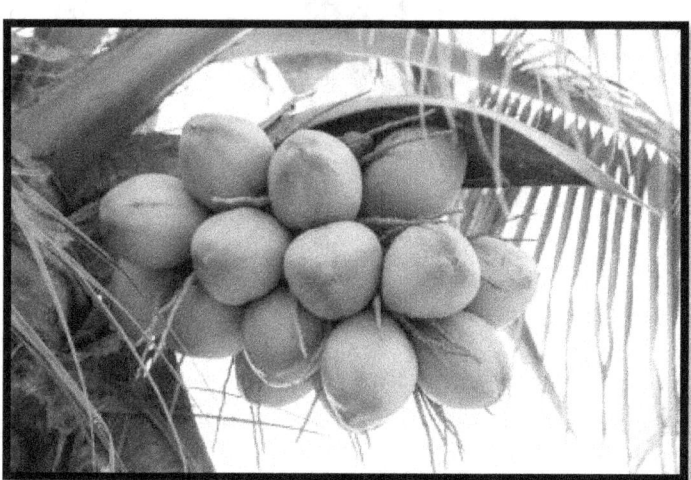

Another interesting feature of coconut is that it reduces the appetite. Management of hunger is very effective for people who are looking to lose some weight by eating less. You can eat coconut and avoid unhealthy snacking habits.

It Can Help With Seizures

The MCTs increase the concentration of ketone bodies in blood; which studies have shown, helps in reducing seizures in children with epilepsy.

Reduces the Risk of Heart Diseases and Enhances Blood Cholesterol Level

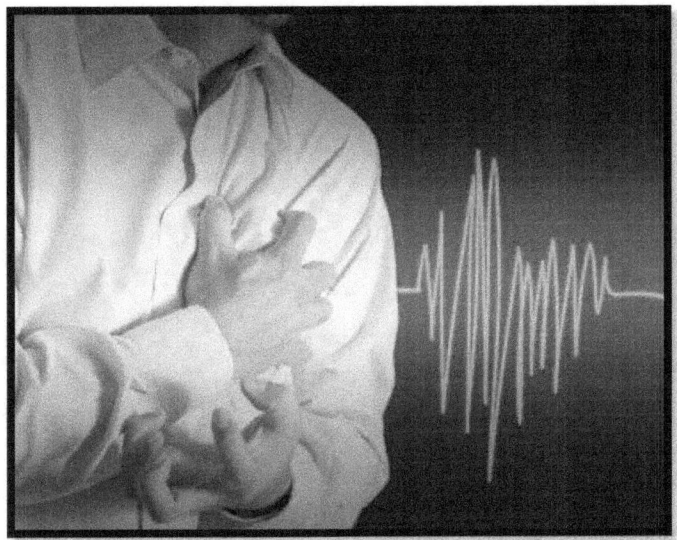

Studies show that coconut oil plays an important role in improving risk factors such as HDL, LDL, and Total Cholesterol levels which may reduce the risk of cardio vascular disease for the people who consume coconut oil in their diet.

It Boosts the Function of Brain Activity and Can Help Alzheimer's Patients

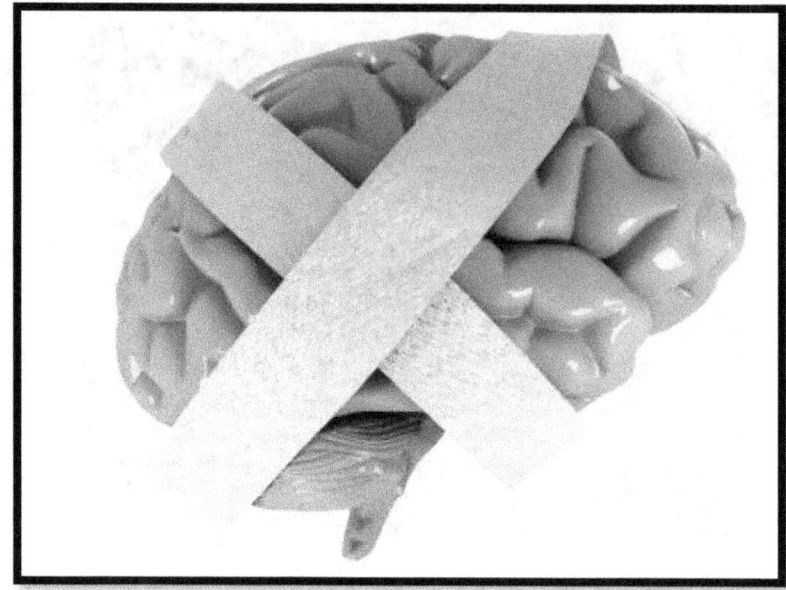

Studies show that consuming MCTs leads to a rapid improvement in the brain function of Alzheimer's patients.

It Helps to Lose Fat, Especially In the Abdominal Region

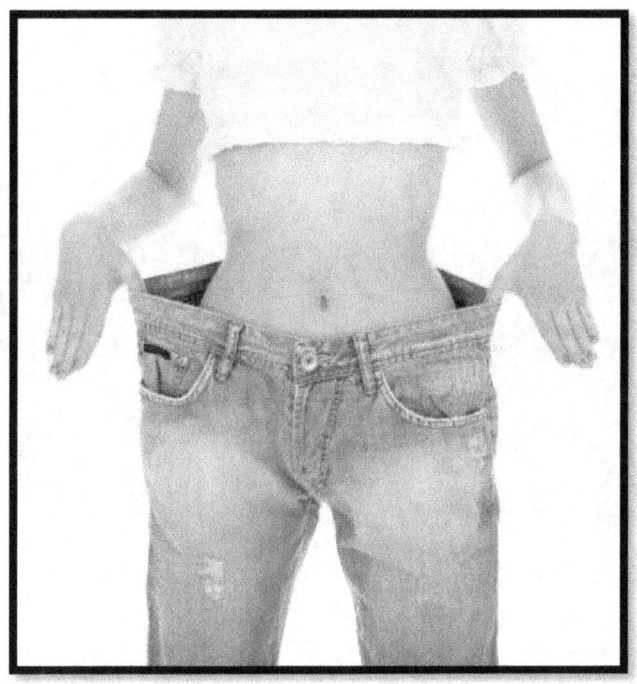

Abdominal fat is the most dangerous of all and can be accounted for as a reason behind a lot of diseases. A study involving 40 women who were given 1 ounce of coconut oil every day showed a significant reduction in their waist circumference and BMI in just 12 weeks.

It Reduces a Person's Susceptibility to Cancer and HIV

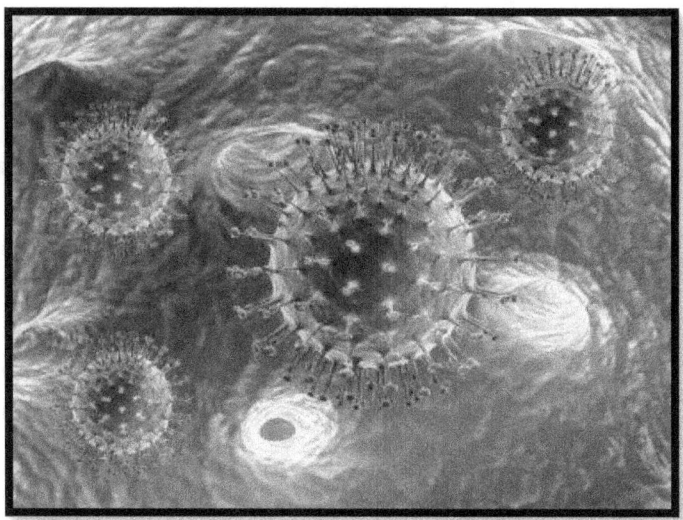

Studies show that coconut oil plays a major role in decreasing a person's susceptibility for viruses, for cancer, and HIV patients. Coconut oil also reduced the viral load in HIV patients in initial research studies.

12 Health Facts about Coconut Oil

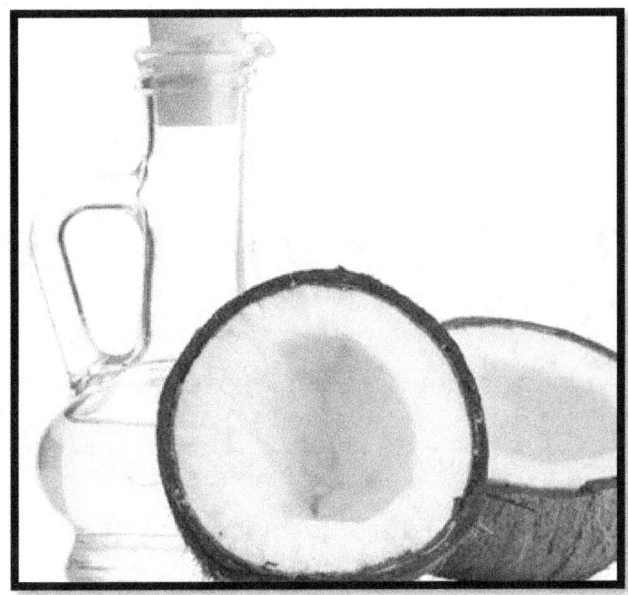

If you haven't been convinced and already decided to start using coconut oil, here are 12 more health facts about it that will definitely make you change your mind.

1. Lauric acid in coconut oil will keep your heart healthy and reduce the risk of cardiovascular diseases.

2. Since it is easier to digest, people who eat coconut and consume coconut oil are not overweight, obese, or fat.

3. It is your one stop beauty product for your hair, skin and nails.

4. MCTs present in coconut oil are an excellent and rapid source of getting energy for body functions.

5. Coconut oil retains its healthy quality even if it is heated at high temperatures and is therefore ideal to be used for cooking.

6. It is also great for vegetarians because it is free from any dairy or animal product.

7. Apart from being heart friendly, it will enhance your immunity towards viruses, bacteria and fungi.

8. It is ideal for Alzheimer's patients as it increase the supply of energy to the brain cells.

9. Since it is rapidly broken down to get energy, it is ideal for athletes or people who do vigorous exercise.

10. It tastes amazing and is great for making desserts as it has a natural sweet flavor.

11. People who have problems of indigestion should eat meals cooked in coconut oil because it is very easy to digest and is light on the stomach.

12. Make sure that you choose unprocessed virgin coconut oil as it contains good fatty acids.

Conclusion

Coconut oil is not only good for your hair and skin; it is equally good for your overall health. It is one ingredient and beauty product that you must have in your house at all times. It not only has a very distinct and natural taste, but it is also very good for your heart and kidneys and also helps in decreasing levels of stress.

It is time that you stop being conned by expensive beauty products and try out this amazing natural product that will make your skin and hair healthier in no time. Plus it is also great for people who are following the Paleo diet or are vegetarian because it is fit for both diets.

So start using this magical liquid today and let it work its magic.

www.ingramcontent.com/pod-product-compliance
Lightning Source LLC
Chambersburg PA
CBHW080342290526
45791CB00009BA/2694